Printed in Great Britain
by Amazon

50022237R00058